Optimization For Athletes: Train For Your Goals, Break Through Plateaus, and Get Results

This book is solely for information and educational purposes and is not medical advice. Please consult a medical or health professional before you begin any exercise, nutrition, or supplementation program or if you have questions about your health.

ISBN: 9781723713699

TABLE OF CONTENTS

Part One:

Weight Training For Results

Introduction: Working Smarter

Would you rather work hard or work smart? I feel both are necessary to achieve greatness, but you can't go far without one or the other. From my perspective, I envision that the end goal is whatever someone is trying to achieve (their goal), which is a pointer to a destination on a map. Working smart is like setting up the compass to go in the right direction, while working hard is actually doing the driving.

You won't go anywhere if you don't work hard, and you'll go the wrong way if you only work hard, because you were not working smart to be able to go in the right direction. However, you might reach your final destination the fastest, if you point the compass in the right direction and move quickly by **simultaneously working smart and hard.** Since you are reading this book, you are probably a hard worker, and this book will supplement your efforts by having you reach your goals in the fastest way possible.

There are many reasons to weight lift. Weight training reduces stress, decreases the risk of injury (for sports and in general), it improves posture, longevity, as well as improve athletic performance. However, not everyone has the time to spend 2 hours in the gym 6 days a week for various reasons such as school, work, social events, sports, and family. In this section, you will learn how to lift based off desired goals, how to periodize your training, and how to optimize your performance; all in as little time as possible. Through reading, you will become better at working smarter; pointing the compass in the right direction.

Phases of Weight Training For Athletes

Some weight lifting coaches and common sports weight lifting programs do not periodize their weight training program. For optimal sport and strength performance, periodizing your training is a great way to get a competitive edge. Periodization is great for athletes because it gives the **best training responses** to those that implement this style of training. Using these phases in a program also gives athletes more results with less time spent in the weight room, so they can focus on their sport.

There are 5 main phases for a weight training program. Generally, the program should last a few months to a year, but is a great fit for a season's worth of time (3-6 months for most sports). **The 5 phases are**:

1. Hypertrophy

2. Basic Strength

3. Strength and Power

4. Taper

5. Active Rest

Phase One: Hypertrophy

During this phase, the athlete is getting adjusted to the weights from a prolonged break (postseason), even if it's their first time of weight lifting. Even experienced lifters should start with this phase if they are starting a new athletic season or just want to hit the "reset button" on achieving new muscle gains. The goal of this phase is to add a bit more muscle to their frame and achieve **nuclei overload**. The nuclei overload is basically adapting the muscles for more *potential* future growth and strength, by keeping a constant stress on your muscles. This future strength will convert towards more speed and power in your respective sport.

This is another reason why athletes that started while young are better prepared to be exceptional athletes when older; they had extra overload of their muscle nuclei from exercising in their youth (i.e. youth sports). However, don't be worried if you did not play sports when you were a kid; you can incorporate this training at any time and achieve superior results when done properly. Remember, the more muscle that is built in this phase, the more potential for future strength.

A great protocol for the hypertrophy phase is to focus on high volume but low intensity training. This means around **3-5 sets of an exercise with 8-15+ reps**, to build up your nuclei. For selecting a weight load, pick a weight where you can comfortably complete 8 reps, but can not perform at 16 reps (failure). This principle follows for any further rep range recommendations.

The more days of the week the athlete lifts (frequency), the more volume they can achieve. This period's length will depend on how much the athlete has trained, and should last a bit longer for newer lifters. This period is usually 2-6 weeks.

The 300 Rep Challenge

After my first swim season in college, my friend, Gabe and I decided to lift for the first time after weeks of tapering in swimming. As we were finishing up our training, we ran into our lifting coach from the season, Parker.

"You guys wanna do some biceps with me before you leave?" he asked.

Gabe and I looked at each other and exclaimed, "Yeah sounds great!"

Parker replied, "Okay we're going to do some bicep blasters!"

"What are bicep blasters?" we asked.

"We're going to do a total of 300 reps of bicep curls, starting with the heaviest barbell. Once you fail at the highest weight, immediately drop to the next highest weight and go until failure. Count your reps and you can't stop until you reach 300. No rest," he said with a maniacal grin and tone.

Gabe started with the 100 pound barbell (he's pretty strong), and I started with the 90 pound barbell. We did as we were told and after a few reps, we dropped the weight. After around 50 reps, we had to rest (with a little bit of ridicule from

Parker). After 100 reps, we had to move to dumbbell curls (DB). At around 250 reps, we had to rest after performing just 5 reps of 5 pounds! It is noteworthy to state that the three of us finished the 300 reps, with our biceps "blasted". However, the next day in class, we couldn't even lift our pencils to take notes, because our biceps were so sore!

This anecdote is an extreme example of hypertrophy type training, but even more exemplifies the nuclei overload of the muscle. Since then, I have barely trained biceps no more than once every two weeks. My biceps have hardly shrunk since then, they respond exceptionally well to any training stimulus, and they have been extremely strong.

It follows back to the principal that the more reps, sets, and days you exercise, the more *future* potential for strength and muscle retention. If you are just starting out or have taken a break for a while, the more reps, sets, and times per week you lift, the better off you will be by the end of your program. For quick reminder, think, "Volume, Volume, Volume!" (Volume=SETS X REPS X FREQUENCY).

Phase Two: Basic Strength

The main focus of Basic Strength is how it sounds; building strength. Since the athlete is to focus on strength, the rep ranges have to decrease with the actual weights increasing. Typical Basic Strength programs fall under 3-5 sets of 5 reps, with 5X5 being very popular. This period is a transition from high volume to medium volume, but bringing up the intensity to the next level. This period usually lasts 3-4 weeks. This is the transitional period from hypertrophy to total strength and power, which will be showcased in our next phases.

Phase Three: Strength and Power

In this phase, gaining strength and not size is the goal. If you are training for a sport, you don't want too much muscle on your frame as it may hinder some speed, so growth should start slowing down at this point to create time to focus on strength. In this phase, more recovery is emphasized, which is not only beneficial for strength performance, but for giving an athlete to focus on their sport training instead.

Going through these phases properly will help you in the long term by *resensitizing* your body for future hypertrophy phases to come. This phase will increase the maximum tension your muscle fibers can handle, which will translate to faster speeds in one's sport.

To increase the strength of an athlete, reps have to be lowered further. This phase is also a time to begin building power; lifting not only with more weight but more *speed.* To gain power, an athlete must decrease the volume of training to be able to recover and become more explosive through safe, controlled movements.

Sets in this phase are generally between 3 and 5, while reps go down further, with 1-3 reps per set. This phase lasts anywhere from 2-4 weeks, depending on your sports' season length. For example, if your season lasts 6 months, this phase should last 4 weeks. If your season is 3 months, this phase should last around 2 weeks.

Phase Four: Tapering

Tapering or "peaking" is the phase that athletes tend to love the most. This is when the athlete should receive massive amounts of rest, with most of the volume cut down. The goal of this phase is to get the athlete used to **exerting maximum force** into the weights, benefiting greatly from lots of rest. This phase is used to adjust the athlete for peak performance, lasting 1-2 weeks. The reason the athlete will become their best self is because of "supercompensation". Supercompensation is basically your muscles adapting from previous training sessions, created from extra rest.

Rep ranges in this period are still between 1-3, but the *volume* drops to as little as 1-3 sets per session.

Fun Fact: The Russian Olympic Weightlifting team loves doing **5 sets of 2 reps**

3x per week is optimal during this period that lasts 1-3 weeks. After tapering, an athlete should feel very energetic, powerful, and ready for their max lift or competition.

How Long to Taper?

A difficult question to answer for weightlifters and athletes all around is, "How long should I taper for?"

This question is asked because if you taper for too long, you "miss your taper" and your muscles and body become deconditioned through not enough stimulus. Essentially, the athlete hit or missed supercompensation from their training. This will lead to poor performance at your final max lifts (or sports competition).

On the flip side, if your taper is not long enough, your body will be too broken down and your body has not recovered in time for your competition, also leading to poor results. While it's hard to tell *exactly* how long you need for taper, there are a few guidelines you can follow.

- **Body Fat %**: If you tend to have a low body fat percentage (under 12% for men and 22% for women), you will need a **longer taper.**
- **Muscle Mass**: If you have a lot of physical muscle mass built up, you will need a **longer taper,** since there is more muscle that needs recovery compared to a person with an average amount of muscle.
- **How you feel**: It's okay to listen to your body. If you are rundown and extremely more tired than usual by the time you reach the taper portion, you will need a **longer taper.**

It is important to be aware of these factors as taper is a **highly individualized** time period where the athlete has to be **truly honest** with how they feel. If you are an individual with low body fat, high muscle mass, and has been training to the ground, you may need this low volume-high intensity period for a **month or more.**

On the flip side, if you find yourself with higher body fat, lower muscle mass, and feel extremely energized during this phase, your taper may need to be as short as **3-7 days.** For each of these factors, **add around 1 week to your taper phase for each attribute you find yourself to fall under.**

Phase Five: Active Rest

This is the hardest phase for a driven athlete; taking a break from training. This phase takes place when the athlete has completed their competition or completed their goals. Be happy and proud you completed the first four phases and/or finished an entire sport season as it is not easy.

If you are really "antsy" to get back to training, take a few days of complete rest, then return to light training. If the athlete is tired in any way, they should take longer rest to completely recover from a hardworking season.

Note: This periodization of phases does not just work well for weight lifting. If you are a coach looking to change up your training, follow these principles for volume and intensity and your team will prosper. If there's one thing to remember from periodization,

- Periodization is to start with high volume, but low weight on the bar.
- As the season progresses, decrease the volume and increase the weight.
- At the end of the season, increase the weight and increase the rest.

Types of Muscle Contractions

There are many ways to grow the strength and size of muscles. You can change your volume (amount of times worked out), reps/sets (# of times you lift a weight), and you can change the intensity of the lift (the load itself).

See, there are 3 main ways you can change the contractions of your muscles for a **shorter, more effective workout.**

The main three ways to contract your muscles are through:

1. Isometric Contractions
2. Eccentric Contractions
3. Concentric Contractions

1. Isometric Contraction: Squeeze the Muscle

An isometric contraction (or isometric hold) is where you are not moving at all, but you are holding the weight at the top or bottom of a movement, contracting your muscles in a safe way. There does not have to be a weight load present for this type of contraction to be effective, so this can be done with any bodyweight exercise. The best example of an isometric contraction is a plank. You are holding the plank through your abdominal muscles and you are contracting them without necessarily moving them. This "hold" will simulate extra reps, without having to perform extra reps.

Isometric holds are also great for building stabilizer muscles; the tiny muscles that protect your ligaments and joint. This is beneficial towards **preventing injury**, as well as **great physical therapy** for problematic muscles.

Our swim team implements isometric contractions for shoulder strength, mobility, and injury prevention. This type of contraction has many practical uses for a variety of goals.

Fun fact: abdominal muscles respond best to this type of contraction.

2. Eccentric Contraction: Lengthen the Muscle

An eccentric contraction happens when the muscle is lengthened. This is usually when you are lowering the weight (depending on the exercise). This contraction extends the "time under tension" of the muscle, which simulates extra reps.

An example of using an eccentric contraction is when you are coming down on a bicep curl. Your muscle gets lengthened at the bottom of the lift as the arm is lowered.

Eccentric contractions develop the most soreness of the three contractions, meaning it is great for muscle growth, but will take longer to recover. Because of the heavy muscle damage, this eccentric contraction may hinder some strength goals, unlike the other two contractions (isometric and concentric). You perform an eccentric contraction by **lowering the weight as slow as possible.**

3. Concentric Contraction: Shorten the Muscle

A concentric contraction is the opposite of an eccentric contraction, i.e., the muscle becomes shortened. This is usually the first thing that comes to the mind of people when they hear "lifting", because it's the actual lifting portion of a movement.

In our bicep example, this is where you curl the weight to the top. At some point in every lift, there will be a concentric contraction, unless you performed a set to failure. There isn't anything "super fancy" about this contraction, because it's just a complicated way of saying the "up" portion of the lift.

How to Use the Three Contractions within Periodization

Back in high school, I took part in the afterschool strength and weight lifting program. It was highly effective; everyone in the sport/club gained strength on some level and most gained incredible strength and muscle. People were increasing their MAX lift by 100 and sometimes 150 pounds in just one season.

After years of research involving studies and training books, not to mention 9 years of lifting experience with various programs, I realized how "Coach Joe", my lifting coach, had such success with lifters of all levels. He had every set, rep, and exercise structured.

He periodized his training with high volume the first few weeks, then gradually decreased the volume towards the end of the season; so, we were well rested for max-out day (finding the most amount of weight we can lift for one rep or "**1 RM**"). We even had a similar 300 rep challenge (shown above) with our biceps on the first day, focusing on high volume and reps (hypertrophy).

Throughout the spring season, Coach Joe would rarely have the same workout twice. If we were doing regular front squats one week, by the next week, we would implement the isometric hold to the front squat by holding the squat at the bottom of the lift for at least 3 seconds. If we were lifting upper body and doing incline bench press, we would slowly lower the weight for about 3 seconds, performing an eccentric contraction. Implementing different contractions helped us grow more muscle and in turn, strength. Before I started training properly, my maxes were as follows:

At 14-years old and no training:

Bench: 135

Back Squat: 225

Deadlift: 250

At 17-years old with 3 years of proper strength training:

Bench: 315

Back Squat: 385

Deadlift: 420

This strength increase over the course of 3-4 years has been attributed to the combination of periodization and various incorporations of muscle contractions. Without them, results would still come, but at a significantly slower rate. This is how I have been able to grow stronger and maintain my muscle mass in as little as **3 hours per week**.

The best time to incorporate variations in your lifts with contraction and periodization is **if you are stalling in your program**. Hold your squats at the bottom of the lift, lower your weights more slowly, or simply add some more reps to add variety and intensity to your training.

These contractions also work well with a partner. A partner can hold the weight against you as you raise your legs to the sky on a leg raise or apply pressure to the bar as you are curling a weight up. There's lots of room for creativity when incorporating different muscle contractions.

The Super Rep

Another efficient way to utilize these contractions is to perform a "super rep"; using each of the contractions in just one rep. To perform a super rep, lower the weight slowly, hold on the bottom, then explode on the way up; all in one rep.

Power (described below) is built from the fast rep on the way up (concentric), extra muscle tension and damage is created as the weight is lowered (eccentric), and during the hold (isometric) at the bottom, there is further muscle damage. This super rep can cover the basis for most strength, size, and power goals.

Lifting For Your Goals

When an individual walks into a weight room, there should be a goal in mind for that training session. Such goals could be: building muscle, burning fat, getting stronger, having more athletic performance, etc. Deciding on which goal you want will determine your training session will help determine what needs to be accomplished and how long you will need to be in the weight room. Some of these goals could overlap, while some can't, or at least not optimally in any category.

Building Muscle

If your goal is to build muscle, high volume is your best friend. This means doing 5 sets or more per exercise, with 5 or more exercises, 5 times a week. Think of 5X5X5 (sets, exercises, and frequency) as an easy reference to building muscle. Generally, more volume=more muscle, with total volume being sets x reps x frequency.

On the diet set of things, be sure you are on a caloric surplus (eating more calories than you burn). Eat around 1 gram of protein per pound of bodyweight, and eat a little more carbohydrates than usual. Creating new muscle tissue is an expensive process for your body, and it's going to be easier if you are eating enough calories. If you don't wish to use a handy app like 'MyFitnessPal', then a good rule of thumb is eat until you are full. **Be slightly fuller more often than slightly hungry** and the caloric surplus will naturally come.

If you still are still having trouble, another useful technique to find how much you need to eat (for growth), is to take your bodyweight in pounds and multiply it by 20.

Examples:

150 Pounds X 20 = 3,000 calories needed to bulk

120 Pounds X 20 = 2,400 Daily calories for bulking

Note: Read more in part 2 of this book for more diet tips

Antagonist Muscles: Build More Muscle In Less Time

A great way to build muscle faster than many lifters is to train opposite or antagonist muscle groups. My favorite exercises for incorporating this style of training is bicep curls with a rope and tricep pushdowns with a rope. The biceps and triceps are antagonistic muscle groups, meaning that as you lift one, the other stretches. As I curl up my bicep during the lift, my tricep becomes stretched and allows it to recover as I am curling. When I push down in the tricep pushdown, my bicep is being stretched.

All that needs to be done is place the pin from the top of the rack to the bottom of the rack or vice versa, saving a lot of time. **Remember, whatever muscle is being exercised/contracted, the opposite muscle is being stretched.**

Other combinations that work well with this principle are:

- **Bench Press and Pull ups**: The chest is stretched from pull ups, while the back is stretched during bench press

- **Leg Extension and Leg Curl**: The hamstrings are stretched during leg extension, while the quadriceps are stretched during leg curl.
- **Dips and Pull ups**: The dips work the lower chest and stretch the traps, while pull ups work the traps and stretch the lower chest

Another way to think about it is to **push for one exercise and then pull for another exercise.** Pulling usually involves using the back side of your body, while pushing involves muscles on the front side of your body.

Remember, this is beneficial for more muscle growth in a shorter training session, as you are performing the sets **back to back**, giving one muscle group some recovery while the opposite becomes fatigued. This greatly saves time because there is no rest when going from one exercise to the opposite exercise.

This is best used for "isolation" exercises such as most machines and "single joint" lifts, as shown in the leg extension and leg curl combo. This is because it is too fatiguing to perform supersets like these with compound movements and other multi joint exercises (ex. bench press, front/back squats, deadlifts).

Note: Do not use this style if you only care about strength as strength is dependent on recovery. Performing exercises back to back dampens recovery in the short term, and you will not be as strong for your compound lifts due to the fast volume build up. **For strength, be at the gym feeling energized.**

Training to Muscle Failure: It isn't always necessary!

You don't want to train to failure if strength is your goal. Our definition of training to failure will be when you no longer can perform any more reps in a set, **without sacrificing form.** When a person loses form, other muscles come in to compensate, defeating the purpose of the exercise.

Training to failure heavily damages the central nervous system, dampening recovery for days or even weeks! Your muscles become extremely fatigued, not to mention the additional soreness that will come! Training to failure should not be done frequently, especially if you are an athlete in a training program.

If strength and athletic performance is the goal, leave a few reps "in the tank" and stop your set before failure. Another problem with going to failure is that your form tends to wane and you start to bring in other muscles into the equation.

So when is the best time for failure?

The best time for training until failure in one or more sets is when you have a few days (3+) before the next time you workout (ex. Vacation, emergency, other responsibilities, etc.). This relates to the central nervous system, because you will then have some time to recover your nervous system by the time you reach your next workout.

Another scenario where training to failure is viable is if your goal is to gain muscle mass and you are in the **hypertrophy phase**. Training to failure is actually a decent way to gain muscle fast if you don't mind being tired occasionally and don't mind training at less than 100% of your energy.

If you are somewhere in between these scenarios and want to occasionally train to failure (which is what I like to do), **try going to failure for just the last set of any exercise in your workout.** This will give sufficient muscle damage, but not to blast your body to the ground. If you want to implement this training technique, I still recommend taking **at least one day off.**

Other Goals

Burning Fat

If your goal is to burn off more fat, you want to be sure to optimize not only your training, but also your diet. Burning fat and dieting are not always for aesthetic reasons. Sometimes an athlete will benefit from some weight loss to fit a competition weight that will feel best for them. An endurance runner will not want to be carrying an extra 10 pounds of fat when they are running over 26 miles; they will (most likely) feel and perform better when they lose the extra 10 pounds.

On the training side of discussion, the goal is to maintain muscle while losing fat. This is not only because muscle is jet fuel for one's metabolism, but also because muscle is a great driver of athletic performance.

The best way to maintain muscle is through consistent training and getting enough protein. To be on the safe side, get around 1 gram of protein per pound of bodyweight (ex. 160 lbs = 160 g of protein). This will ensure you hold on to your athletic performance while simultaneously reaching a comfortable competition weight.

While you may be able to build muscle without being in a caloric surplus all the time, you **absolutely** have to be in a caloric deficit to lose fat. This caloric deficit will force you to sacrifice volume, because energy levels are much lower during a caloric deficit.

Sets should stay around the number 5, with the exercises staying around 5 as well, but only *if* you lower the days per week to as low as 3 days per week (5 sets of 5 exercises 3 times a week). **Something in terms of volume should be sacrificed** the longer you stay in a caloric deficit, with the consequences being extreme burnout if you continue with high volume. If you are looking for a simple formula that is fairly accurate, take your bodyweight in pounds and multiply by 10. This will be the calories to eat each day to lose fat.

For example, if you are 200 pounds, 2,000 calories will be a great amount to shed some fat. Burning fat is a massive topic that can become extremely complicated under different conditions, so stay focused on the things that matter and **keep lifting and getting your protein.**

Building Muscle and Burning Fat at the same time: Can you do it?

There is a small fraction of the lifting community that could burn fat and build muscle simultaneously. The best candidates for this position are those that have just started lifting, those that have not lifted in a few months, the gift of genetics, and those on steroids. The reason these populations could simultaneously burn fat and build muscle is because their muscle building response is so great; they could build muscle in a calorie deficit.

Remember This: A caloric surplus simply **helps** muscle building, while a caloric deficit is a **requirement** for fat loss. Training is the biggest driver in muscle gaining. And while training helps fat loss, you can overeat the calories you burned through training with just a few hundred calories (3 pieces of fruit) and undo your fat loss efforts.

A simple way to think of these goals is to eat more to gain muscle, and eat less to lose fat.

Modified Reverse Pyramid Training: A Program for Strength

When my goal is to achieve strength with a little bit of muscle growth on the back end, I implement my own version on reverse pyramid training. Here's an example first with an explanation after.

Bench Press (or any **compound** movement):

Set 1 (warm up): 20X135

Rest: 30 s

Set 2 (Heaviest): 3X275

Rest: Unlimited

Set 3 (2nd Heaviest): 4X260

Rest: 3-5 minutes

Set 4 (3rd Heaviest): 5X250

Rest: 1-2 minutes

Set 5: 8X225

Do you see what is happening here? After a quick warm up set, I immediately start with my heaviest set. This will focus on my type 2 muscle fibers or "fast twitch" muscle fibers to grow strength, speed, and a little bit of size. As I go through more sets, I increased the reps and lower the weight, hence the "reverse pyramid" part of the name. By the time I am on my last set, in this case set 5, I am less focused on strength and more focused on muscle contractions; feeling the mind connect with the muscle.

This is further exemplified with **the rest decreasing throughout the sets, giving the muscles less time to recover and in turn, more muscle in less time.** This is why it's a "modified" reverse period because most reverse pyramid training programs do not incorporate both strength and size.

Lifting for Strength and Power

Lifting for strength and lifting for power are similar in some ways and different in others. Strength training is focused on lifting as much weight as possible, in any way possible, while power training is more finessed. Power training needs to be incorporated for all athletes *on some level,* as it is what will increase the **explosiveness** of the athlete. However, explosive movements can be implemented to almost any lift or bodyweight movement to turn it into power training. For example, you could take the back squat and add an explosive jump at the top of the movement, building speed in the athlete's legs. Here are some guidelines with a chart.

Strength Styled Sets:

5 sets of 3 reps at 80% of 1RM

Power Styled Sets:

5 sets of 8 reps at 60% of 1RM- **with a jump**

Here is a chart that can help distinguish the two:

Strength vs. Power Training Properties

Strength Training	Power Training
Overcoming resistance	Overcoming resistance
Heavy weight (75%+ of 1RM)	Any weight
Contributes some muscle gain	Lifting **as fast** as possible
Moving **from point A to B** the easiest way	Plyometrics and other body weight exercises benefit

Optimizing Your Performance: "Hacks", Tips, and Tricks

How to Breathe During Exercise: Understanding which part of your breath is best for each point in your lift

Scientific research has shown that strength increases by about 5% when you clench your teeth, when you clench your fists, and when you breathe correctly during exercise.

Knowing how to breathe during your lift would take your strength to the next level. Did you know that you are strongest when your breath is held, a little weaker when you exhale, and are at your weakest when you inhale?

This means at the **bottom** of your lifting movement (ex. Bottom of a squat, the bar touching your chest on bench press, etc.), you want to **hold your breath**. This is because you are naturally your weakest at this low point so you have to compensate by holding your breath. **As you come up** from the lift, the bar feels lighter and lighter, so **exhaling your breath is the most beneficial**. As you come down in the movement of your lift, you should inhale so as to prepare for holding your breath as the lift becomes harder and harder.

As a quick summary, **remember this:**

- You are strongest when you hold your breath
- You are a little weaker when you exhale
- You are weakest when you inhale

Give this a try right now! Take a deep breath and hold it... Don't you feel powerful and strong? That is how you will feel underneath the bar. Now exhale. What did you feel? You may have experienced your body relaxing as you exhale. Pay attention to your breath from time to time. **You will discover that it is a huge factor in many daily activities** in decreasing stress, falling asleep faster and deeper, and ultimately being in control of your day.

Warming Up: It's not just to get you tired

I used to think that the more I warmed up, the more tired I was going to be during the main training portion; so, I admittedly didn't warm up well with my sport teams. Most people know the importance of warming up and how great it is for optimizing performance, but I was too stubborn to actually try to properly warm up. Since then, I have researched and experimented many times over, with and without warming up and how my performance responded to it. The results? Warming up can make or break your performance.

The internal temperature of your muscles can greatly affect your performance. Did you know that for every 2 degrees Farenheit your internal temperature is raised, your body can become up to 7% stronger? This is because the mitochondria in your muscles perform best when your body is just a few degrees above its normal state, with blood being able to flow easier.

If you're not carrying around a thermometer (like most people), the best way to know you finished warming up is when you have just **started to break a sweat**. At this point, your body is primed for optimal performance at its best body temperature without getting yourself fatigued, and you may experience that 7% increase in strength.

Nitric Oxide

Another reason warming up will enhance your performance is blood flow. When your body has more blood flow, your body creates something called nitric oxide. This is a very **good** thing. **Nitric oxide** expands the blood vessels, increases blood flow, decreases plaque growth, increases blood clotting, and opens your muscles to intake more nutrients. So if you want to get the most benefits and nutrients from your food, be sure to warm up at least until you break a sweat.

Breathing through your nose is another easy and simple way to boost nitric oxide. The next time you warm up, **try to perform all or most of the warm up by only breathing through your nose.** Give this tip a try while you are walking somewhere or doing anything. This will boost the overall oxygen in your blood over time in a natural way.

There are some foods that can boost nitric oxide. Here's a list to add to your grocery cart:

- Watermelon
- Bananas
- Spinach
- Seafood
- Garlic
- Dark Chocolate (the darker the better)
- Lemons
- Grapefruit
- Walnuts
- Oranges
- Rhubarb
- Apples
- Strawberries

- Beets

Fun Fact: Beets are my favorite food to boost nitric oxide naturally in the body.

Sleep: Sometimes doing nothing is better than doing something

Have you ever had to wake up early in the morning day after day for school, work, or sports? As a hardworking lifter, athlete, or both, you deserve your sleep. In fact, you should make sleep a priority, especially as you progress further into your training.

The longer and deeper you sleep, the more Growth Hormone (GH) you will release. Growth Hormone is the ultimate anti-aging hormone, destroying inflammatory free radicals that are created from daily stress and exercise. This means you are literally slowing down time (in terms of your body) the more that you sleep and increase how long you can live. Growth Hormone will also help grow healthy hair, skin, and nails; it isn't called "beauty sleep" for nothing.

Rest is just as important as training. However, this does not mean that you should sleep 12 hours a day or sit on the couch for hours. Rest compliments training just as training complements resting. The more you train, the more rest you need to compensate for training; like a teeter totter. Rest is where the adaptations and growth occur *from* your training. Sadly, most people do *not* rest enough and become burnt out and quit their activity.

The best way to get deeper, more restful sleep is to have a sleeping mask. The sleeping mask will create a dark (almost black) atmosphere in almost any environment. This dark environment helps your body produce melatonin; your main sleep hormone. This happens extremely fast and your mind will wander less and less. This saves hours of tossing and turning and will get you to sleep faster so you can take on your next day of training with full energy.

Training Template: Strength

Shown below is a great training template that can be mixed and matched with the list of exercises (listed later).

Lower Body

Exercise	Sets	Reps	Rest	Intensity/ Weight
Deadlift	3	4	Unlimited	High
Step ups (weighted)	4	6/Leg	90 s	Med–High
Squat Jumps	3	8	60 s	BW
Bulgarian Split Squat	3	5/Leg	90 s	High
Plank	2	90 sec	30 s	BW

Upper Body

Exercise	Sets	Reps	Rest	Intensity/ Weight
Bench Press	5	5	60-120 s	High
BB Bent Over Row	4	6	90 s	Med-High
Shoulder Press	3	6	60 s	High
Lying Triceps Extension	3	5/Arm	90 s	High
Clap Push ups (knees if starting out)	3	6	45 s	BW and ALL OUT

Note: If you are focusing on strength, you need to decrease the reps and sets but increase the weight. The 'rest' noted in this section is extremely variable, since everyone is in a different cardiovascular condition. It is advised to remember that when training for strength, you are to rest until you feel almost at 100% energy. Don't go into a set breathing heavily with an extremely high heart rate; it will defeat the purpose of the workout.

Training Template: Muscle Growth

Lower Body

Exercise	Sets	Reps	Rest	Intensity/ Weight
Back Squat	5	6	60-90 s	Med-High
BB Single Leg Squat	4	8/Leg	60 s	Med-High
DB Calf Raises	5	20	30 s	Med
DB Lunge	3	8/Leg	90 s	Med-High
Wall Sit	2	90 sec TUT	60 s	BW

Upper Body

Exercise	Sets	Reps	Rest	Intensity/ Weight
Incline Bench Press	5	8	60-90 s	Med-High
Pull Ups	5	8	60 s	Med-High
DB Curls	4	8/Arm	60 s	Med
DB Shrugs	3	20	30 s	Med
Bicycles	3	60 s TUT	30 s	BW+Contract hard

Note: If your goal is to gain physical muscle size, volume is key. Focus on contracting and *feeling* the muscles and you will reach your optimal size before you know it.

Training Template: Power Training Exercises

Full Body

Exercise	Sets	Reps	Rest	Intensity/ Weight
Power Clean	5	4	Unlimited	Med-High
Standing Shoulder Press	4	6	90 s	Med
Good Morning	4	8	30 s	Low-Med
Box Jumps	3	8	60 s	High
Medicine Ball Throws	2	6	30 s	Med-High
Battle Ropes	2	30sec TUT	90 s	All Out

Note: Power cleans are amazing for building speed, power, and explosion. It is **horrible** for muscle growth since the eccentric and isometric portions are almost nonexistent.

List of Weight Lifting Exercises and their Benefits

The templates above are just general guidelines to follow and the exercises are not as important as the volume and intensity associated with them. Feel free to mix the template with any of the exercises shown below for your desired goal. My notes following the exercise are the way I use the exercise, but you can manipulate the volume and intensity for your goals.

Chest

- **Incline Barbell Bench Press**- Great for gaining general strength and some upper chest development
- **Flat Barbell Bench Press**- Great for gaining strength and mid-chest development

- **Incline Dumbbell Press**- Great for growing muscle in the upper chest and evening out the strength in your arms
- **Flat Dumbbell Bench**- Evening out strength in arms to create more balance and strength for the Barbell bench press
- **Dips**- Developing the lower chest and rarely used for strength
- **Cable Crossovers**- Development of the inner chest
- **Incline Chest flys**- Great for development of the upper chest
- **Medicine Ball Throws**- Builds power and recruits fast twitch muscle fibers in the chest

Shoulders

- ***BB Shoulder Press (standing)-** Best compound movement for the growth of shoulders with additional use of the abs and back for stabilizing the body
- **BB Shoulder Press (sitting)-** Higher weight can be used for more strength of the shoulders since you don't have to stabilize your body
- **Seated Dumbbell Press**- Evening out strength and size of shoulders

- **DB Lateral Raise-** Developing the outside of your shoulders, with the weight pivot getting heavier towards the top of the movement
- ***Cable Lateral Raise-** Similar to the dumbbell version, but a constant *linear* tension throughout the movement
- **Face Pull-** Developing the trapezius and upper back muscles
- **Dumbbell Front Raise-** Developing and growing the front of the shoulders (*Usually this muscle group is not a problem for most people as it tends to get overdeveloped through incline and flat bench press)

Back

- **BB Deadlift-** Great for total body strength, athletic performance, and overall muscle development (*lengthy in set up and tear down of weights)
- **BB Row-** Great for developing *thickness* in the back
- **Dumbbell row-** Great for evening out the strength and size of the back muscles
- **Pull Ups-** Best all-around exercise for the back for strength and size. Wide grip for more lat development and close grip for more focus on shoulders
- ***Chin ups-** The only compound movement for your biceps

- **Lat Pulldown**- Great for developing and focusing on just the lats
- **Shrugs (BB or DB)**- Best development for the traps

Abdominals (Abs)

- **Planks**- Implementing the isometric hold and building stabilizer muscles
- *****Bicycles**- Fast breakdown of your abs and my favorite exercise to get in great ab work in a short amount of time
- **Leg Lifts**- This could be done on many pull up machines as well. Targets the lower abs.
- **Russian/Roman Twist**- Works the serratus (upper side abs), especially when weight is used.
- **Incline Sit Ups-** A great total ab contraction through extra range of motion compared to traditional ab exercises

Legs

- *****BB Back Squat**- Best "bang for your buck" lower body exercise for strength and development of your hamstrings (backside of thigh)
- *****BB Front Squat**- Another great lower body exercise for development of your quadriceps (front of thigh)

- **Leg Press**- Best machine for pain free squatting that is great for starting lifters, taller people, or people with rough joints in pain
- ***Lunge (BW, DB, or BB)-** Great compound movement for development of the legs that can be done anywhere
- **Leg Extension**- Machine great for quads (be sure not to go too heavy or you may have joint issues)
- **Leg Curl**- Machine great for your hamstrings
- **Box Jumps**- Builds power in the legs

Arms

- **BB Curl**- Best curling exercise for strength
- ***E. Z. Bar Curl**- The jagged bar helps with keeping your joints comfortable with full range of motion
- **DB Curl**- Great for general bicep development
- **Hammer Curl**- Great for developing the length of your bicep (front portion of bicep)
- ***BB Close Grip Bench Press**- Great for developing the triceps and inner chest and is the best compound movement for your arms
- ***Triceps Pushdown (rope)-** A great exercise for developing mass in your triceps (back of arms) that has a constant tension that is linear throughout the lift

- ***Bicep curl (rope)**- Great for immediately after the tricep pushdown as an antagonist muscle (see above) and for constant linear tension for even development over other curl-type exercises
- **Battle Ropes**- Great explosive work for the arms and builds cardio for longer periods of time under tension

Notes:

favorite of mine = *

DB= Dumbbells

BB= Barbells

If you noticed some trends from the exercise list, **the most important things to remember are:**

1. Barbells: Focus on strength
2. Dumbbells: Evening out strength on both sides of your body
3. Cables and Ropes: Focus on muscle growth and provides linear tension as opposed to variable tension from barbells and dumbbells.

Tools and Supplements

There are a few main supplements that help sports performance. Most other supplements (not shown below) are usually a waste of time as they are either filled with banned ingredients, don't work at all, or can actually hurt you. These supplements I recommend below are the safest and develiver the best "bang for your buck" (benefits to cost) that help sport performance.

Creatine Monohydrate

Creatine is naturally produced by the body but you can also get it through your food. Some foods that contain creatine are shrimp, beef, chicken, and most other types of meats. You can also get creatine in supplement form which is the form of creatine that is most practical for noticing a difference in performance.

Creatine helps your performance by allowing water (and other nutrients) to rush into the muscle cells and swell up. This allows for greater strength and speed for lifting and high intensity sports. Sadly, some people are non-responders to creatine, so it's important to check to see if creatine will even work for you.

Creatine will give you greater training adaptations and muscles growth in less time. Think of creatine as a "muscle hydrator" that keeps your muscles filled with water and nutrients for a longer period of time. In turn, you will be able to lift more and train harder each day, which will results in greater muscle damage and strength. While creatine *indirectly* helps athletic performance (for the reasons stated above), it does not magically build muscle if you are not training hard enough. You can **not** just sit around on the couch all day and build muscle. Use creatine to *supplement* your training and don't rely on it as the *base* for your training.

You can start with a dose of **about 5 grams per day,** which is usually just a teaspoon from most supplement bottles. If you are noticing a bit more strength in the next few weeks, you respond well to creatine. Stick with creatine monohydrate, as it is the most researched supplement among the supplement industry.

Whey Protein

Another great supplement for your performances is whey protein. Remember when I mentioned earlier that you should get one gram of protein per pound of body weight? Whey protein could help you here.

There are 3 main types of whey protein:

1. Isolate
2. Concentrate
3. Hydrolysate

1. Isolate: This contains 90+% protein by weight, with low fats and low carbs and lactose removed and moderately priced.

2. Concentrate: This contains 30-90% protein by weight with the rest being carbs and fats.

3. Hydrolysate: This contains extremely broken down protein that is extremely digestible but is the most expensive

All of these different types of protein will help your lifting and athletic performance by helping you achieve that 1 gram of protein per pound of body weight recommendation. If you want the best bang for your buck, concentrates and isolates will be the best options for you, as they are cheaper than hydrolysate.

If you tend to have an upset stomach (from isolate, concentrate, or just in general), whey hydrolysate will be your solution. However, the training adaptations you receive will be very similar or the same among these 3 types of whey.

Protein will be the best tool to help your muscles recover and grow back stronger. Think of whey protein as convenient protein to be used to *supplement* your protein needs when you can't cook or are "on the go".

Coffee/Caffeine

I am a huge fan of coffee. There's something about it that just puts me in a great mood along with a motivating feeling to do more work each day. I also use coffee for sport and lifting performance.

Caffeine is a stimulant that affects the nervous system. Remember when we were discussing the nervous system breaking down when training to failure? The nervous system breaks down if it becomes extremely overtaxed, with a recovery period long enough to drain your energy for days to even weeks. Caffeine will stimulate your nervous system, with the more that is consumed, the more your nervous system becomes taxed. Some reasons for a corrupted nervous system are overtraining, too much stress, not enough sleep, and too much caffeine.

So why have I recommended coffee? Doesn't coffee contain caffeine? In times like this, it's always good to remember, the dose of something determines the *poison* of something. Caffeine in high amounts will make you feel as I like to say, "Wired and tired," so, we need to find the correct dosage for ourselves. Coffee does not contain too much caffeine and 1-2 cups offers a comfortable dose. Don't drink too much, as you may start to develop a **tolerance** (see tolerances and sensitivities in part 2).

To test your tolerance, take 1 cup at a time each day and find the point where you have a moderate amount of energy without your heart beating out of your chest. What I find is best for lifting is no more than 1-2 cups of coffee, but what works best for me may not work best for you, since I have a weaker tolerance than my peers.

If you don't like coffee, you could try pre workout supplements or energy drinks. However, they are a slippery slope because your body quickly adapts and then depends on them *just to feel normal.* I'd recommend mixing only a small amount in your water bottle, so you are mostly hydrating yourself; getting a smaller kick of caffeine in the background.

If you have this light dose of caffeine, you are stimulating your nervous system just enough to activate the "fight or flight" response in your body to move with maximum power and speed; something that will greatly help your lifting.

If there's one thing to remember from consuming caffeine to help your performance; **smaller is better**. You should rely on your training, nutrition, and a good warmup as your base for performance. Drink 1-2 cups of coffee to *supplement* your training.

Fun Fact: Caffeine is a banned substance by the NCAA, but only in an amount of about 8 cups (600-1,000 mg of caffeine) of coffee (consumed around 2 hours before competition). This is why a pre-workout supplement is not a great idea, due to caffeine content upwards of 240 mg per serving. You wouldn't want that amount of caffeine anyways as it does not help performance and could give the user a heart attack during exercise (in extreme cases).

MCT Oil

MCT oil is a supplement but almost considered not a supplement. MCTs or "medium chain triglycerides" can be found in coconut oil, which means it is part-food. "Triglyceride" basically means just fat; the only macronutrient in MCT oil. However, MCT oil itself is a supplement because it is usually extracted from coconut oil or manufactured in a lab.

MCT oil is a great energy source for activities that are in the mid-distance range where the time a person is exercising is between 30 and 60 seconds. As in the name, it is a medium chain triglyceride, not a short or long chain triglyceride like butter or other fats. This fat bypasses the liver when eating, meaning it almost instantaneously gives you energy. Just 1 tablespoon will produce a burst of stable energy lasting around 1-4 hours.

If you are nervous about trying MCT oil, give coconut oil a try! It has around 40% MCT oil in it, along with health benefits of "lauric acid" to help with inflammation and recovery from workouts. I'm no coconut oil guru, but I have found coconut oil and MCT oil helps me generally feel great. For training, there tends to be noticeable boost of **endurance.**

Energy Sources During a Set

When you are lifting and performing a set, your body is using different types of fuel as the intensity or reps are manipulated. The energy system corresponding with the reps below being **only accurate if the last rep is failure or 1-2 reps shy of failure.**

Reps 1-3: You are using the creatine phosphate system

Reps 4-15: You are using the anaerobic system

Reps 15+: You are using the aerobic system

The Creatine Phosphate System

Earlier, I mentioned creatine as a supplement for increasing speed and strength. The creatine phosphate system is the reason creatine gets a shout out. During the first few seconds of any intense exercise, in this case reps 1-3, you are **using your creatine stores.** Earlier, I mentioned that there are some foods that contain creatine such as meat and seafood. While these foods do replenish your creatine stores, you can't always keep up with the demand. Those foods, unless eaten in large quantities, only offer 2-3 grams of creatine. This is where supplementation comes in (5 grams per serving) if you want to train hard and recover hard.

Fun fact: Usually the first hard and fast movement you do anytime and anywhere involves using creatine and its phosphate system.

The Anaerobic System

In a rep range of 4-15, you are starting to tap into your anaerobic system. This system is also used in sprinting. For the anaerobic system, "time under tension" (TUT) or time you are exercising is around 15 seconds up to a minute. At this intensity, a great amount of sugar (glucose/carbohydrate) is being used, so go ahead and allow more carbohydrates in the diet. A great sport that utilizes the anaerobic system is American football, sprinting on and off in repeated intervals. You will use this energy system the most when lifting.

Remember: Think of any intense movement that lasts longer than 10 seconds as you using your anaerobic system and eat more carbohydrates.

The Aerobic System

At 15 or more reps (or TUT over around 1 minute), you are using the aerobic system. As the distance in an endurance event increases, you are forced to use more of your aerobic system, because the lower intensity needs to be maintained longer . At this intensity, contrary to popular belief, fat is your best friend. Fat is your friend when you go the distance (or do lots of reps) because of fat being slow digesting, giving a steady state energy longer than the crash carbs can give.

Note: For more information on energy sources, intensities, and even body types, read on to part 2.

Part Two:

Macronutrients For Performance

Eating For Fuel

An athlete should train and eat differently if they are a powerlifter versus an ultra-marathoner, but there needs to be a difference in training and nutrition even within the same sport (ex. sprint swimming versus mid distance versus long distance swimming). Knowing these variances can make all the difference from getting a record to not being able to improve at all to becoming worse at one's sport.

Both in and out of season, an athlete should be aware of any and everything they put in their bodies. Each food and drink that goes in has a different response in the body for every athlete, with food combinations creating even more complicated reactions. For example, did you know if you eat a grapefruit with coffee, you make the caffeine in the coffee last longer with less of a crash? This is because grapefruit has a compound called "naringin", that is shown to extend the half-life of coffee. Knowing "hacks" like this has made huge differences in my athletic career in speed, power, and recovery.

If an athlete is reaching for fast food and packaged snacks and goods without thinking about it, they are not reaching their full potential.

"But have you heard that Usain Bolt eats chicken nuggets before his races?" People have told me.

First of all, Usain probably has a contract deal with McDonalds, so he's going to say what he needs to say to help promote McDonalds and its brand image. Secondly, even if he does eat chicken nuggets, he probably does not eat them all the time or every day, like many athletes in the United States and around the world do. Lastly, even if he does eat Mcnuggets all the time every day, think of how much faster he could be! Just because he is the fastest human alive does not mean he could not be even faster *without* the nuggets. Correlation does not mean causation, and this part sorts out much of the research over the years that helps lead us to the truth.

The swim club that I coach has an annual lake swim in one of the many lakes of Minnesota, where the coaches swim with the athletes. After the lake swim, we shared breakfast together and I had an interesting conversation with one of my coworkers who was swimming with me.

She swam for the University of Miami and made it to the Olympic Trials in the 400 Meter IM and the 200 Meter backstroke. She was a very high level athlete. I asked her what her diet was like in her prime and the diets of the swimmers around her, to gain further insight to sort out all the "mumbo jumbo". She emphasized many lean proteins, lots of veggies (but only after a workout or competition, not before), and even a little bit of red wine on some nights (*if you are of age).

She told me about her taper and what the diet was like for her and her collegiate friends: they would start "carb loading" around two weeks prior to the championship swim meet. This carb loading was very incremental and small, as opposed to shoving all the carbs in the house into your mouth. These means they slowly increased the percentage of carbs of their daily total calories and ate at maintenance calories to not gain or lose weight (more on carbs and calories later).

She even spoke about how they would not eat any dairy products at least 48 hours before competition to avoid any digestion or stomach issues. On competition day, they ate very little or nothing, because all their energy was stored from the carb-load two weeks prior. They were able to have a better blood flow and a better race because their stomachs were not tied up in digestion of large amounts of foods.

This short anecdote gave some common insights and shows that the top performing athletes pay close attention to their diet and nutrition. However, in this portion, we can take an even deeper analysis of nutrition. To play and compete with high level athletes, we should be just as aware, if not *more* aware than these athletes.

MACRONUTRIENTS
We can't live without them so why not understand them?

Carbs

Carbohydrates are usually the quickest way to get some fast acting energy that is best for sprints and other high intensity exercises. If an athlete is depleted (just trained/exercised), they will be more receptive to take carbohydrates into their muscles as energy to store for later than if they had not just trained or had just eaten carbs. Carbs come with a price, however. After depleting your carb stores or "glycogen", the muscles release a higher amount of lactic acid than if you were to eat a meal higher in fat. This is not totally bad, but it increases the need for a longer recovery before the next intense movement. Eat fewer carbs if you can't afford to crash (ex. three more quarters left, multiple events at a meet, or longer styled events >30 seconds).

Think of getting candy stuck in your teeth. That sugar from the candy sticking to your teeth is the same way sugar/carbs (all carbs convert to sugar once digested) stick to your muscles and sometimes restrict blood flow and even air flow. However, this happens on a very small scale and most of the time is not noticeable. If you are an endurance athlete but you can't sacrifice carbs in the diet for whatever reason, there is a *temporary* solution.

Have you seen marathon runners gulping down drinks like Gatorade and PowerAde during the actual marathon? They are constantly refueling their glycogen stores just as they get depleted. This is a temporary solution because their body will end up relying too much on the carbohydrate for energy and will develop a tolerance (see "Tolerances and Sensitivities"). In addition to this tolerance requiring higher intakes of non-nutritious sugar, if there is no sugar available, they may even go hypoglycemic and feel faint (or actually faint). This means this technique works great only when the endurance athlete is sensitive to carbohydrates from slightly cutting them down a few days prior to competition. Otherwise, stick to carbs working for you rather than against you and read further.

Fats

Fats, in the world of athlete diet recommendations, tend to get pushed in the back behind carbs. They are usually recommended in small amounts and not talked about enough. However, many athletes dominate competitions off a high or higher fat diet than the traditional diet.

Remember how I asked you to imagine candy getting stuck to your teeth? Think of oils and how tough it is to stick them to anything and how it would be impossible for them to stick to your teeth. Now think of olive oil or coconut oil in your hands. It's very moisturizing, smooth, and a great skin therapy.

When fats are eaten and burned in your body, it is a very smooth and even source of energy. This is because fats slow down the digestion of any meal as a whole and are slow to digest themselves. It gives an athlete a stable and *long* source of energy for hours. This stable energy is great for mental performance in any work, school, or job situation.

As with all these macronutrients, fat has its downsides. Because of fat's stable energy, it's tough to get high and intense bursts of energy and power from fat. If an athlete tries to buffer this by eating more carbohydrates with the fat, the athlete may get a bit sleepy. This is because carbs release serotonin, a relaxing hormone. When combined with fat, the fat adds density to the meal, requiring heavy digestion, making you even sleepier than before. This effect is proportionate to the meal size, meaning more food will make you sleepier. Think of how you feel after a massive Thanksgiving dinner and you feel like falling asleep and taking a 3 day nap. Combining fats and carbs in a small meal is the same effect as that Thanksgiving dinner on a smaller scale.

What you should do as an athlete that wants or needs both carbs and fat and reap the benefits of both is to separate your fats and carbs throughout the day.

For example, my college swim team has two practices a day and sometimes I want the benefits of fat to get me through the practice, but I also want to be able to sprint for practice, utilizing the carbs stored in my muscles. I will wake up, and if I'm hungry I will have a few eggs (cooked any way), then I will swim from 6am-8am. I will then have a whey protein shake with unsweetened almond milk after practice (no carbs yet). If I am still hungry for lunch, I will have a few vegetables with some low fat yogurt, adding a little bit of carbohydrate with a lower fat content. I will swim in the afternoon from 3pm-5pm and then have dinner.

Dinner consists of higher carbs and higher protein (see nutrient timing) and medium fat. I can afford the extra fats and carbs because as the day comes to an end, I *want* to be a little sleepy. For a bedtime snack, I will eat anything left to fill my daily requirements. This layout enables me to train with a light stomach and receive a great adaption to the training from the heavier meals later in the day.

This may sound tedious but it really is not. It is simply being a little more aware of what is being put in the body and how it affects the body. This is valuable because once you understand proteins, carbs, and fats, and how they interact; you can control your energy for the day.

Protein

So what's the deal with protein? Why have I saved it for last?

Protein is the macronutrient that should be manipulated for weight loss and training demands, *not* for weight gain or even extra athletic performance. That is, protein intake should be *raised* if the goal a person has is to lose fat. Because a calorie deficit is needed for weight loss; fats, carbs, or both fats and carbs should be lowered to create this deficit. Losing weight is sadly horrible for athletic performance, *unless* the athlete is extremely overweight and needs to get to their ideal competitive weight. This competition weight varies from athlete to athlete and can only be best determined by whether they feel good or not at their current bodyweight.

So, what should we do with protein? We simply just need to **eat enough of it.** Protein rebuilds any broken tissues in the body and clumps together amino acids that in turn build muscle. This muscle gives athletes more power to work with in their sports and more importantly, greater nutrient storage. The more muscle, the more chances food goes into those muscles, as opposed to your fat cells. This is because muscle makes you **insulin sensitive**, meaning it helps your pancreas shuttle nutrients more effectively.

I find that as long as you don't drop below 60 grams of protein a day, you should not see your muscle mass drop.

Ideally, however, an athlete who is a sprinter should aim for around 1 gram of protein per pound of bodyweight per day (ex. 160 pounds should strive for 160 grams of protein per day). Protein needs decrease a little as the distance increases, but don't fall below .5 grams of protein per pound of bodyweight (80 grams if 160 pounds). This is because the high intensity of sprinting usually results in a higher protein breakdown compared to other intensities, and needs to be replenished so to compensate for this breakdown.

Athletes that stick to these guidelines can find that it is actually pretty expensive, and sometimes a little too filling, to meet their daily requirement, as protein is the most expensive macronutrient and the most filling one, with fats following next in line. Don't worry if you don't always get your protein requirements (1 gram/pound). There won't be much of a difference in terms of muscle growth or muscle mass unless the athlete is hungry all the time or hardly ever eating any protein. You don't often want to go higher than this one gram per pound of bodyweight anyways due to protein sensitivity (See Tolerances and Sensitivities).

HIGH-CARB VS. LOW-CARB

The debate continues

I am a sprinter. I have always sprinted from high school football, to track and field in college, to swimming in college. Sprinting almost exclusively requires glucose; sugar or carbohydrate. When I first learned this, I was always doing my old version of "carb loading"; simply shoving in as many carbs as possible as frequently as possible. This is not the definition of carb loading but I thought it was because I was never told the strategic approach. Big mistake. Not only did I not get any extra athletic performance for my intended goal of sprinting, my weight went through the roof and I was 230 pounds at 5'7.

The only thing this extremely high carb and high calorie diet will do is make you very heavy, but at least you will get very *strong*. My one rep maxes for my weights before going high carb were as follows:

Bench: 205
Back Squat: 275
Deadlift: 315
@180 LBS at 16-years-old

After my high carb and calorie diet:
Bench: 315
Back Squat: 385
Deadlift: 420
@230 LBS at 17-years-old

As you can see, my strength increased immensely. You could even go as far to say that mostly coach Joe was the biggest factor in this strength, discrediting carbs on some level. But how were my sprint times?

50 yard freestyle: 24.6 s
100 yard freestyle: 52.3 s
@180 LBS at 16-years-old

Which led to:
50 yard freestyle: 32.9
100 yard freestyle: 1:02.1
@230 LBS at 17-years-old

So what do we do? Well one of the biggest things I have found watching high level sprinters compete that was not obvious to me was that when it comes to performance and food, especially carbs, *moderation* and maintaining a *lower body fat %* were two consistent factors throughout most sports.

The fastest sprinters have the lowest body fat while maintaining a glucose metabolism; basically meaning their bodies performed and felt best off of carbs over fat. This poses another problem for someone who is overweight and runs better off of fat. What I mean by "better off of fat" is that you tend to get more energized from dietary fat or your body fat itself, from eating more fat and less carbs for a few weeks. If you run better off of fat, your sprint performance may decrease. Adjusting your macronutrient ratios will have food work in your favor rather than against you.

Ultramarathon runners; how do they not bonk? They run hundreds of miles each week and are pretty good at it. They rely more on the utilization of fat. See, the molecule for dietary fat (the fat that you eat) is similar to the body fat on your body! One may think that this is bad, and in some cases it is. In some cases it isn't. Fat, both dietary and the fat we wear, is best burned at low intensities. Because the exercise is low intensity, the athlete will be able to use it for longer periods of time before burning out. If the athlete runs out of dietary fat (the fat we eat), the body efficiently switches to running off its own Since fat has 9 calories per gram (as opposed to 4 calories per gram in carbs and protein), it is almost impossible to run out of unless you didn't eat anything for weeks!

The longer the distance, the more intensity that has to be sacrificed. The time where more sugar may be needed for a marathoner (or ultra-marathoner) is when the intensity increases, which makes your heart rate increase. A situation where this may happen for a marathoner may be when they speed up to pass the runner next to them, sprinting down a hill, or sprinting to the finish line. At times like this, a sport drink may be helpful, as the extra carbohydrate will aid this intensity.

What helps clear out the confusion is a simple heart rate chart.

Heart Rate Chart

Age	Max HR	50%	75%	80%
20	200	100	150	170
25	195	98	146	166
30	190	95	142	161
35	185	93	138	157
40	180	90	135	153
45	175	88	131	149

If you are like me and don't like memorizing chats, a simple formula is 220-AGE for your MAX heart rate. After that, it's easy to "guesstimate" the percentage. As an example, let's say you are 21 years old.

MAX HR = 220 - (21) = 199 or ~ 200
At 50%: ~100 BPM: you are burning fat for fuel and carbs won't help much

At 75%: ~150 BPM: you are burning a pretty even mix of fats and carbs

At 80%: ~170 BPM: you are burning mostly carbs here. Eat more carbs

At 95%: ~190 BPM: you are only burning carbs at this intensity. Be sure to have adequate rest if this intensity is to remain

I don't use the heart rate system that often because perceived effort and how tired something makes me feel is often a pretty good indicator of what fuel source I am using. For example, if I am out of breath with a high heart rate, I know I am burning more carbohydrates.

Another easy tip to think about this concept is the higher the % of intensity (or perceived effort), the more carbohydrate you will be using. The lower the heart rate and intensity, the more fat you are burning (dietary or body fat). For example, when sleeping, the intensity is pretty low; about a heart rate of 40. This means that when you are sleeping, you are mainly burning only fat molecules because of its low intensity being only 20% (give or take) of your max heart rate.

On the alternative side of things, if you were out in the wilderness and a wild (angry) grizzly bear snuck up on you, you may go into a dead sprint as fast as your legs will allow you to go. Let's assume that you are running at 100% intensity, because who wants to get slashed and eaten by a grizzly bear? You will only be burning glucose during that sprint.

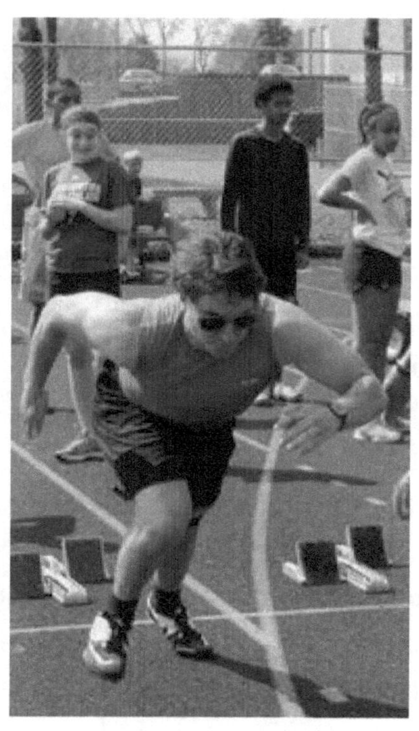

The unfortunate consequences of not eating enough carbohydrates when you absolutely need it is "gluconeogenesis"; the breakdown of proteins to sugar. This could be just be random amino acids (broken protein bonds) throughout the body, but in some cases, it means muscle. Have you ever been extremely hungry during a practice or competition? Well if you have not eaten enough carbohydrate during this time of high demand, your body may start breaking down muscle tissue that is so hard to build up in the first place. This poses a heavy problem for athletes that are not matching their diet with their training. If a sprinter goes low carb to try to shed some fat and they are sprinting frequently (burning lots of glucose), they will start to lose their muscle mass and, in turn, their athletic performance.

I like to have precision in my diet the week before, and especially the night before, a competition. If I have the 100 Meter dash and the Javelin throw the next day, the week and night before that day I will eat mostly carbs, very little fat and moderate protein due to the events having a high intensity type nature. If I wish to maximize my Javelin throw performance, then I will be in a calorie surplus, since the extra weight will only help my throw rather than hurt it.

I will be in a calorie deficit if I care more about the 100 Meter dash, since the slight weight loss will keep me light on my feet and fast. In both cases, I will have the maximum glycogen to perform at these higher intensities of 90%+ of my maximum heart rate. Glycogen is just a fancy word for "stored sugar" in the liver and muscle cells, and is a combination of water and carbohydrate bonded together. Glycogen is a powerful energy source, but is limited as to how much muscle an athlete has and how many carbohydrates they can tolerate and stomach.

If I want to maximize performance in both the 100 Meter dash and the Javelin throw (which is usually the case), I will eat high carbs but keep the total calories for each day at maintenance (I won't gain or lose weight from my diet). If more information is needed about what may or may not be a surplus, find a BMR calculator online and add calories burned through exercise to your BMR (basal metabolic rate) calculation to find out how many calories are needed to maintain your weight.

Base Your Intensity With Perceived Effort

At mid intensity or mid distance cardio, you are going faster than a walking pace but not yet at the level of a sprint (all out). The perceived effort of this jogging speed is medium intensity, assuming you could continue the pace for a while, but not for hours. Fat and carbohydrate are burned pretty evenly at this mid-level intensity, so it is advantageous to eat a diet balanced between fats and carbs.

The specific numbers are not as important as you may think, so just be sure to eat some healthy fats and some healthy carbs and not have too much of one or the other. I like to have a balance of fats and carbs loaded prior to competition for events where I am "under tension" or exercising for *more than* 30 seconds. Shown on the next page is a photo of John Stoltz, swimming the 200 yard breaststroke, a mid-intensity type exercise, burning both fats and carbs throughout the race.

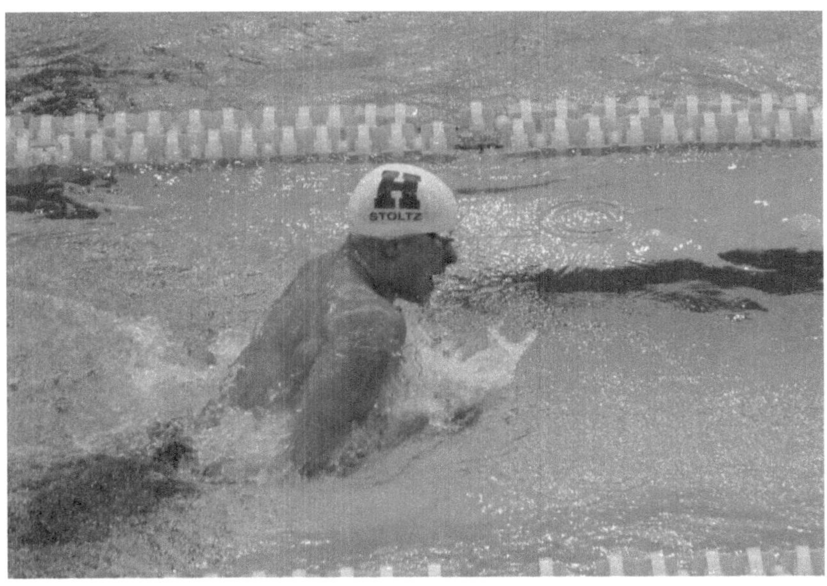

It is important to note that everyone is different. Some people may perform better in distance events with a bit more carbohydrates than the average distance athlete and sometimes a sprinter may sprint or lift more or sprint better with a bit more fat than the average sprint athlete. Causes in these differences are genetics, a person's body type, and their eating preferences throughout their lifetime.

While it is tough to explain how a person's genetics and prior dietary choices contribute to these variations, it is important and simple to understand different body types to find the best diet for not only their sport and event, but for their anatomy.

THREE MAIN BODY TYPES
What do you think you are?

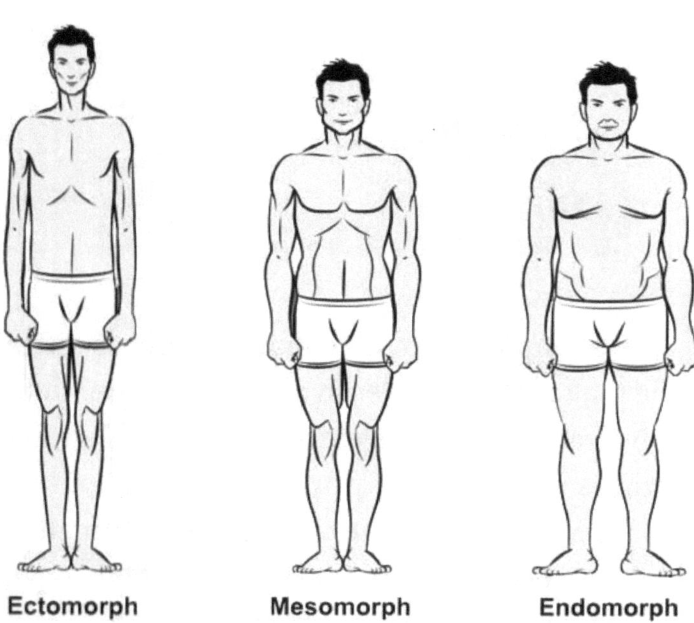

Ectomorph

Have you ever talked to a person who seems to have a "freakish" metabolism? They claim that they have a huge appetite and can eat whatever they want and as much as they want and they don't gain weight—whether it be fat or muscle. They tend to be underweight and very fidgety. These are the traits of an ectomorph body type.

For a naturally occurring ectomorph type of body, **carbohydrates** tend to be their friend in optimizing athletic performance. This thin and lanky body type tends to be very effective at utilizing glucose for exercise and cognitive functions. People that fall under this body type tend to have a bit more trouble digesting fats or running off their own body fat. Load up on the carbs and stick to only healthy fats if you find yourself as an ectomorph.

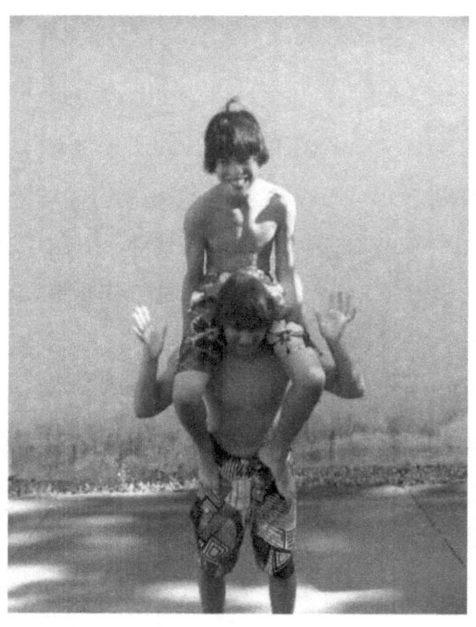

Shown above is a photo of my friend Ed (top) and me (bottom), at 11 years old. As you can see, Ed was a clear ectomorph and I was an endomorph (explained later).

Mesomorph

Over the summer I was coaching a club swim meet for swimmers throughout Minnesota to qualify for the big state swim meet. It was interesting to look at the different body types and what events those body types tended to excel at. On the club I coached, there was a seven-year-old boy named Ricky (name changed for confidentiality). Ricky had almost no body fat. He had a bulging six-pack that most teenage boys do not have, as well as many other muscular features that were not typical of his age.

"There's no way this kid lifts weights!" I thought, "He's not getting this muscle from swimming alone either. In fact, he has missed over half the practices this summer!"

Ricky dove off of the blocks and demolished the competition of the average-developed seven-year-olds in the 100 Meter freestyle, dropping almost 30 seconds and placing in the top 50 in the nation. Meet the mesomorph body type.

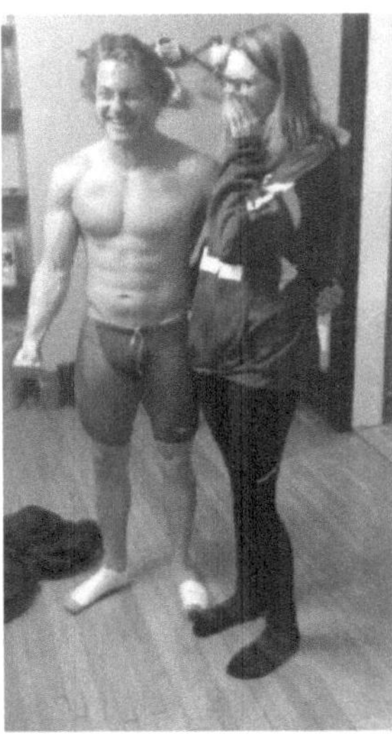

This body type is a desirable body type for most athletes, simply because it is the most versatile. Mesomorphs tend to build muscle very easily, burn fat very easily, and usually have a small waist but broad shoulders. An example of a mesomorph that took advantage of their body type and pushed it to the limits is Arnold Schwarzenegger, one of the greatest bodybuilders of all time.

Weightlifting and sprint style competition are what mesomorphs tend to excel at. Because they are so efficient at burning fat and building muscle, they are able to use both fats and carbs very well. While this efficiency is great, mesomorphs can't utilize carbohydrates as well as the ectomorph or utilize fats as well as the endomorph.

If you are a mesomorph, a balanced diet of healthy fats, carbs, and protein will be the best for this athletic body type. I have seen great athletes both skinny and large, but most of the best athletes are either naturally a mesomorph or they worked hard in the weight room and their sport to *become* a mesomorph. Or at least look like one.

Endomorphs

Endomorphs are the heavy and strong types of athletes. These are usually the throwers in track and field and the defensive or offensive linemen in football. While endomorphs usually have trouble losing fat, they are the best body type for building and maintaining muscle.

Some endomorphs can sprint very fast, especially if their "time under tension" (TUT), or time they are exercising, is *less than* 30 seconds. This is because of the endomorph's ability to put on large amounts of muscle quickly, with muscle being a huge driver of speed in very short sprints.

If you are an endomorph, the best diet for your performance will be high fat, medium to low carb, and moderate protein levels. An endomorph body type tends to run better of fat more than they tend to excel at distance events, due to the extra weight in fat and muscle they have to carry. This is another reason this body type is not optimal for sprints above 30 seconds.

However, there are some pretty noteworthy marathoners that are endomorphic, and they are able to beat out a lot of their ectomorph and mesomorph competitors, showing that your genetics are not an end all be all. This is mostly because if the endomorph runs out of glucose, they have many reserves to tap into with their body fat because of the body's preference for it while an ectomorph may have to rely on something sugary to keep them going.

NOTE: An endomorph tends to gain body fat faster the more carbohydrate in their diet, so it is important for the endomorph to keep track of how insulin sensitive they are by watching their weight in response to more or less carbs in their diet.

Optimal Starting Macronutrient Ratios

<u>Sprinting Macros:</u>

60% Carbs

25% Protein

15% Fat

<u>Mid Distance Macros:</u>

50% Carbs

25% Protein

25% Fat

<u>Distance Macros:</u>

30% Carbs

25% Protein

45% Fat

Body Type Macros

<u>Ectomorph Macros:</u>

60% Carbs

25% Protein

15% Fat

<u>Mesomorph Macros:</u>

40% Carbs

30% Protein

30% Fat

<u>Endomorph Macros:</u>

25% Carbs

30% Protein

45% Fat

The reason I don't lay out these macronutrients in grams is because I don't know how many calories you need. Amount of exercise, bodyweight, genetics, hormones, sleep, metabolism, and even factors like how fast you eat affect total calories needed. To help clear possible confusion, let's say you burn 2,500 calories based off the BMR calculator. Let's assume you are an ectomorph and your sport requires a medium intensity most the time so your macros are:

40% Carbs

30% Protein

30% Fat

This would mean that you need:

250 grams of Carbs

185 grams of Protein

83 grams of Fat

The best app to track this is MyFitnessPal. It allows you to set the percentages of your macros how you like along with a calorie goal and gives you the numbers you need to perform optimally. Using this app is much more accurate than simply guessing and estimating your macros and calorie intake.

These three body types are not set in stone. These body types are the guidelines and are a **spectrum**, and anyone can fall anywhere on that spectrum. Me, for example, I am an endo-mesomorph; I am somewhere between an endomorph and a mesomorph. These principles laid out hold pretty true to me as well; I can easily gain and keep muscle, perform a bit better on a slightly higher fat diet than a mesomorph, but have a tougher time losing fat in addition to an easier time gaining fat.

Wherever you think you fall on the spectrum, start with the recommendation I lay out for your macros, and slightly adjust as needed until you feel optimal. Finally, adjust your macronutrients again for the type of exercise you wish to excel at.

For example, an ectomorph may naturally run better off carbs but if that person with the ectomorph body type wishes to do endurance events (fat based), they will want to start with a moderate carb, moderate fat, and moderate protein diet, since endurance-style events call for a higher fat diet. The way this is calculated is by taking an average of the macros I recommended. In my example above, the endurance-ectomorph needs:

(60+30)/2= 45% Carbs

(25+25)/2= 25% Protein

(15+45)/2= 30% Fat

This formula is a great way to align your food with your biology and optimize performance.

Top Foods by Category for Optimal Athletic Performance

Fats- endurance based, >30-60 seconds	Proteins- maintaining and building muscle	Carbs- sprinting, weight lifting, <30 seconds
Olive Oil- great monounsaturated fats and best used in salads uncooked	Chicken- cheap and versatile	Sweet Potato- packed with vitamins with no energy crash
Grass Fed Butter- high amount of healthy fats (omega 3)	Egg Whites (or whole if desired)- slow digesting and a lean source of protein	Regular Potatoes- higher initial energy than sweet potatoes with a small crash
Avocado Oil- the superior olive oil and can be cooked at a high temperature	Salmon- great amino acid profile: (get more bang for your buck)	Rice- white rice on training and brown rice on non-training days for digestion
MCT Oil- fast digesting fat with no taste	Cottage cheese- Great for before bed! (Slow digesting protein)	Berries- blueberries, strawberries, raspberries, etc.
Macadamia Nuts- I snack on these during the competitions	Whey Protein- simple and easy to add to smoothies or other recipes	Kiwis- more potassium than a banana

Fats	Proteins	Carbs
Coconut Oil- Has up to 40% MCT oil	Greek Yogurt- great for smoothies and before bed	Any Vegetable- stick to carrots or spinach before training for digestibility
Avocados- long lasting steady state energy.	Bone Broth- Pure protein and used by many professional athletes for a high amount of electrolytes	Rice Cakes- easy on the stomach and a great snack for on the go athletes (which is all of them)
Unsweetened Almond Milk- A better tasting milk that is non-dairy	Grass fed beef- one of the most nutritious sources of protein with a slightly higher fat content	Oats- Easy and fast to make. Versatile with many healthy ingredients
Coconut flakes- a great snack that is almost exclusively fat content	Shrimp- almost pure protein and very easy on the stomach, with a few grams of creatine content	Beets- delivers a boost of nitric oxide that improves blood flow for hard working muscles
Dark Chocolate- contains natural stimulants that boost energy (the darker the better)	Pumpkin Seeds- offer a moderate amount of protein and acts as a great snack, with more minerals than most food	Popcorn- the best snack to get in some carbs with a moderate toll on the digestive system (eat only after workouts to be safe)

Tolerances and Sensitivities

Our bodies have different sensitivities to different things; training, proteins, fats, carbs, and even sleep. You want to switch this up around different periods of time to keep all your sensitivities up. For example, if you were sleeping consistently less than 8 hours for even more than a week, the next time you will be able to sleep in, do it! You will find that you may sleep until noon when going to bed at 10pm: a total of 14 hours! If you are eating many carbs for many days, the next week or so, add some fats to the diet and lower the carbohydrates.

Your body wants to always pull you towards homeostasis: where it is most comfortable. If you eat too much protein, your body gets used to the high demand and will need more protein over the long run to perform its functions, similar to an alcoholic who needs more and more alcohol to get drunk.

These tolerances hold true for carbs, fats, and even stimulants like caffeine. This is why I don't choose my macros until a week before competition; when I find out my events for the weekend. Once I know my events, I can eat more carbohydrates or fats for the week, depending on the length of my events. Working smarter and not harder just takes a little bit of experimentation on the body to find what makes you feel the best, and to find the point where you don't develop dietary tolerances.

NUTRIENT TIMING
When is almost as important as what

There is an optimal time to eat each of the macronutrients. As you have learned, your goal heavily depends on what macronutrient needs to be eaten at certain periods. If you focus on timing, it will also help with your tolerances and sensitivity to each macronutrient. The general rule of thumb that helps with most styles of training and body parts is **low carb in the morning and as the day progresses you raise the carbs and lower the fat,** with protein held constant throughout the day.

This allows you to train with low insulin, a hormone released from carbohydrate. This low insulin keeps you *sensitive* to the carbs that are eaten at night, becoming more efficient at storing the carbohydrate in the muscles. Since carbs release serotonin, it is even beneficial for a better sleep. If you are looking to get specific:

- Before an endurance practice lasting more than an hour you should eat: high fat, medium protein, low carb keeping the volume light
- After the endurance practice: low fat, high protein, high carb as a heavier meal
- For before a sprint workout (or lifting) where you will be sprinting less than an hour of practice: medium carb, medium protein, low fat

- After a sprint workout: high carb, medium protein, wait 30-60 minutes then medium fat as a heavier meal
- If you don't know your practice ahead of time, which is usually the case: before, medium carb, medium protein, wait 30-60 minutes then medium fat keeping it light
- After: high carb, high protein, wait 30-60 minutes then medium fat as a heavier meal.

If you noticed the trend, another rule of thumb is to keep a very light stomach the more sprints that are involved and eating a heavier meal if there is a longer duration of activity. This is to help keep optimal blood flow and digestion during your exercise, while still eating enough to not lose energy. Remember, you don't want to be stuffed then have to run repeated sprints and you don't want to go hungry if you are swimming miles at a time.

Training on a lighter stomach also makes you more receptive to the nutrients after the workout, and is a powerful way to prevent tolerances, since you have not eaten as much and the training furthered glycogen depletion. After the depleted state, your muscles act as a sponge and "soak up" extra carbohydrates to be used for their explosive performance.

Notice how I also did not give calories or grams in nutrient timing. This is because everyone has different levels of hunger or definitions of "high medium and low". But for the number oriented person, here are some guidelines:

Low fat: <10 grams

Medium fat: 10-30 grams

High fat: 20-50 grams

Low Carb: <10 grams

Medium carb: 20-40 grams

High carb: 40-80 grams

Low Protein:<10 grams

Medium protein: 20-30 grams

High protein: 30+ grams

Remember these are on a per meal basis and NOT the daily requirements.

If, for whatever reason, you can't count the grams or amount, **eyeballing the amounts is still better than throwing your nutrition out the window.** These can also be adjusted based off your body type because they are great baseline numbers. As mentioned earlier, you may feel better off of higher or lower amounts of carbohydrates, fats, and proteins, so be sure to slightly adjust until you feel great all the time.

Closing Thoughts

Spread the word about this information as it is not commonly told to people. Many athletes and average gym goers (which are athletes) do not go into the gym with their goals in mind, aimlessly getting in a "work out". Apply the training styles and training tips laid out in this book and you will achieve strength, athletic performance, and muscle mass faster than the rest of your competition.

On the diet side of performance, make sure to eat for your event and your body type. This will be a massive competitive edge as most people do not dial in their nutrition. Be sure to eat carbs for sprints, fats for distance, and enough protein to spare your hard earned muscle.

If you have received value from this book, leave a comment and a rating! For more feedback or questions, email me through my business email: breheimgregory@gmail.com

I am still early in my writing career, so I hope to learn what was good or bad and what to work on so that it could be improved on in subsequent future writings. I would also like to hear what you would like to know for future book topics. Take the next step and use this knowledge into your next competitive season and optimize your performance!

About the Author

Greg has participated in a variety of sports and worked with many athletes at many different sports clinics in swimming, weightlifting, football, and track and field. Having competed in numerous weight lifting tournaments, Greg is also a swim coach for the St. Croix Swim Club (2018), one of the most competitive clubs in the midwest. He is a huge fan of trial and error to find some of the best techniques for optimization for each given scenario, constantly learning at each opportunity.